BEDSIDE MANNERS:

A COMPENDIUM OF PHYSICIAN RELATIONSHIPS

Rob Tenery, M.D.

Leonard J. Morse, M.D.,
contributing editor

Cover by Gene Blakeney and Janet Tenery
Photographs by Nell Dorr
Front cover image of Robbie Tenery
Back cover image of Dr. W.C. Tenery and Dr. R.M. Tenery
Photograph on Dedication Page © 2014 Estate of Pablo Picasso/Artists Rights Society
(ARS), New York

ISBN: 1493571052
ISBN 13: 9781493571055

Library of Congress Control Number: 2013920442
CreateSpace Independent Publishing Platform
North Charleston, South Carolina

Dedication

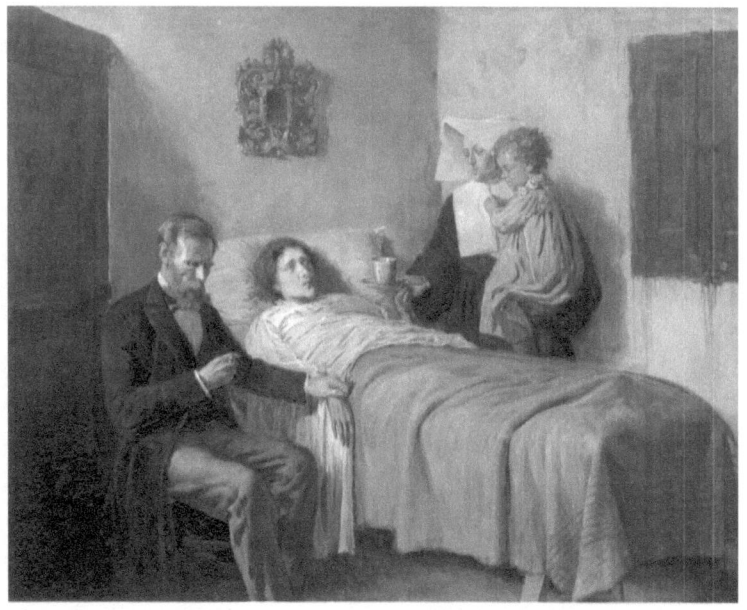

'Science and Charity' Pablo Picasso, 1897

To Dr. W. C. Tenery, Dr. R. M. Tenery, Dr. Leonard J. Morse, and all those physicians who believe the practice of medicine is their calling.

Foreword

Oath of Hippocrates

I swear by Apollo the physician and Aesculapius, and Health, and All-heal, and all the gods and goddesses, that, according to my ability and judgment,

I will keep this Oath and this stipulation—to reckon him who taught me this Art equally dear to me as my parents, to share my substance with him, and relieve his necessities if required; to look upon his offspring in the same footing as my own brothers, and teach them this art, if they shall wish to learn it, without fee or stipulation; and that by precept, lecture, and every other mode of instruction,

I will impart a knowledge of the Art to my sons, and those of my teachers, and to disciples bound by a stipulation and oath according to the law of medicine, but to none others.

I will follow that system of regimen which, according to my ability and judgment, I consider for the benefit of my patients, and abstain from whatever is deleterious and mischievous.

I will give no deadly medicine to any one if asked, nor suggest any such counsel; and in like manner I will not give to a woman a pessary to produce abortion. With purity and with holiness I will pass my life and practice my Art.

I will not cut persons laboring under the stone, but will leave this to be done by men who are practitioners of this work. Into whatever houses I enter, I will go into them for the benefit of the sick, and will abstain from every voluntary act of mischief and corruption; and, further, from the seduction of females or males, of freeman and slaves. Whatever, in connection with my professional service, or not in connection with it, I see or hear, in the life of men, which ought not to be spoken abroad,

I will not divulge, as reckoning that all such should be kept secret. While I continue to keep this Oath unviolated, may it be granted to me to enjoy life and the practice of the art, respected by all men, in all times. But should I trespass and violate this Oath, may the reverse be my lot.

"My doctor is really good," a friend recently said. Contrast this to another comment: "My doctor must be good." The former statement is positive, while the latter conveys a lingering doubt. Both quotes connote a continuing ownership in the relationship. In the latter, the doctor has failed to make a connection and the patient is looking for reassurance. If the physician's competence is also in question, patients often look elsewhere. The bridge to make that connection is what is called the "art of medicine." This art, which takes the relationship to a higher level, is often referred to as the physician's *bedside manner.*

The term *compassion* is frequently used to describe this art of medicine. Caring not just about the malady, but caring about the patient. Caring that they do not suffer, caring that they do not recover alone, and caring that those who love them are also suffering.

Compassion without outwardly demonstrating that sensitivity is without meaning. The art is being able to show this higher level of involvement. It is a willingness to be more than just a scientist by giving of one's self rather than just acting as a "peddler of pills." It demonstrates an investment in one's patients and not just in what is wrong with them. The ability to practice this art is often the single most important factor that elevates one physician above another.

The art is more encompassing than just showing compassion. It is about showing respect. It is about remembering that each physician is also a representative of the medical profession—those who have gone before and those who will come after. It is not just about commitment to one's patients, but to the patients of others as well. It is an appreciation of being part of the medical profession.

The art is also about the ability to adjust and sometimes even compromise to achieve the "greater good." It is taking the time to look above the fray, trying to anticipate and prevent future problems using past lessons as guideposts for future decisions. It is about accepting responsibility, not only for one's patients but also for the whole of the profession. It is an awareness of what it *really* means to be a physician.

This book is a primer on conduct for those who have dedicated their lives to this profession and for those who follow. Even though social norms may change over time, certain aspects of physician behavior remain inviolate.

As growth in the science of medicine moves doctors further away from the "bedside," it becomes increasingly important to remember the general principles of selflessness and compassion that formed the basis of the medical profession's earliest written codes of conduct, earning physicians the respect and trust of their patients and their peers.

FOREWORD

When the American Medical Association (AMA) was established in 1847, the two overriding principles the founders of the organization championed were ethics and professionalism. In 1803, the English physician Thomas Percival published *Medical Ethics*.[1] The AMA representatives used this work to model their first code of ethics. Although revisions to Percival's code have been made by the AMA in 1903, 1912, 1947, 1994, and 2001 to adapt to the changing times, the major concepts and similar wording still remain.

American Medical Association's Principles of Medical Ethics[2]

Preamble—The medical profession has long subscribed to a body of ethical statements developed primarily for the benefit of the patient. As a member of this profession, a physician must recognize responsibility not only to patients first and foremost, as well as to society, to other health professionals, and to self. The following Principles adopted by the American Medical Association are not laws, but standards of conduct which define the essentials of honorable behavior for the physician.

I.   A physician shall be dedicated to providing competent medical care, with compassion and respect for human dignity and rights.

II.   A physician shall uphold the standards of professionalism, be honest in all professional interactions, and strive to report physicians deficient in character or competence, or engaging in fraud or deception, to appropriate entities.

III.   A physician shall respect the law and also recognize a responsibility to seek changes in those requirements which are contrary to the best interests of the patient.

IV.   A physician shall respect the rights of patients, of colleagues and other health professionals and shall safeguard patient confidences and privacy within the constraints of the law.

V.   A physician shall continue to study, apply, and advance scientific knowledge, maintain a commitment to medical education, make relevant information available to patients, colleagues and the public, obtain consultation, and use the talents of other professionals when indicated.

VI.   A physician shall, in the provision of appropriate care, except in emergencies, be free to choose whom to serve, with whom to associate, and the environment in which to provide medical care.

VII.   A physician shall recognize a responsibility to participate in the activities contributing to the improvement of the community and the betterment of public health.

VIII.   A physician shall, while caring for a patient, regard responsibility to the patient as paramount.

IX.   A physician shall support access to medical care for all people.

About the Author

Rob Tenery, MD, FACS, is a past chairman of the Council on Ethical and Judicial Affairs of the American Medical Association, and a clinical professor of ophthalmology at the University of Texas Southwestern Medical School. He is the author of *Dr. Mayo's Boy: A Century of American Medicine* and *In Search of Medicine's Moral Compass*. He is a commentator on his web sight *Echoes for the Future* as well as a clinician and medical historian.

About the Contributing Editor

Leonard J. Morse, MD, FIDSA DSc (hon.) is a past chairman of the Council on Ethical and Judicial Affairs of the American Medical Association, as well as a professor of clinical medicine, family medicine, and community health at the University of Massachusetts Medical School and Graduate School of Nursing. He is a retired commissioner of public health for the city of Worcester, Massachusetts.

Contents

How physicians apply medical science depends on the availability of their resources, location of their encounters, and their individual skill sets. How they incorporate the art into these encounters depends on their devotion and sensitivity not just to the scientist in them but also their personal devotion to those who are in need. Listed throughout the chapters are not dictums but rather observations gathered over of a lifetime devoted to the healing arts. Hopefully, they will serve as gentle reminders that without involvement, physicians are little more than highly paid medical workers.

Patient/doctor relations share commonality with any relationships with similar goals. The same negative reactions of disrespect, outbursts, mood swings, and anger produce similar results. The difference is the imbalance of influence the physician holds over the patient. This advantage should be respected and never abused.

———

Doctors, dressed up in one professional costume or another, have been in busy practice since the earliest records of every culture on earth. It is hard to think of a more dependable or enduring occupation, harder still to imagine any future events leading to its extinction.
—*Lewis Thomas, MD, author, poet, and educator, 1913–1997*

———

1.

Interactions with Patients

The Fashionable Doctor

If you come across a fashionable doctor, watch him carefully at a safe distance before handing yourself over to him. He may be a good doctor, but in very many cases he is not.

First, because as a rule, he is far too busy to listen with patience to your long story.

Secondly, because he is inevitably liable to become a snob, if he is not already, to let the Countess pass in before you, to examine the liver of the Count with more attention than that of his valet, to go to the garden-party at the British Embassy instead of to your last-born, whose whooping-cough is getting worse.

Thirdly, unless his heart is very sound he will soon show unmistakable signs of precocious hardening of that organ. He will become indifferent and insensible to the suffering of others, like the pleasure-seeking people around him.

You cannot be a good doctor without pity.

—Axel Munthe, Swedish psychiatrist, 1857–1949

The patient/doctor relationship is based on the four ethical principles of *autonomy*, *justice*, *non-malfeasance*, and *beneficence*. It is the process of sharing one's knowledge and skills with another in need. In the beginning, there was no formal contract. Instead of a handshake, the offer was a helping hand. The ultimate goal was one of good, and not for any reward that might come out of the encounter.

The relationship was an unwritten covenant between the physician and the patient. It was based on trust. Trust that the physician would always put the patient's best interests first. Trust that the physician would use his or her skills to apply the best diagnostic and therapeutic options available or refer the patient to where those alternatives would be available. Trust that the physician would never abandon the patient.

Then things changed. The physician had to "make a living." What was once a relational union between the physician and the patient began to slowly evolve into one based on a transaction—an exchange between two consenting parties. Those patients who couldn't afford to offer anything in return still received proper care. Those with the means to pay more did—the exchange of skills and knowledge for whatever the receiving party could afford. In those early days it could have been a bushel of corn or a prized farm animal. Later it was more often currency. In spite of this evolution to a transactional relationship, the covenant between the doctor and the patient still stood firm—at least until third parties became involved. At first, it was private health insurance (later to become Blue Cross/Blue Shield) and the federal programs (Medicaid and Medicare). Even then, the covenant was not tested until the federal programs started dictating how much the physicians should be paid (allowable charges).

The growing threat of repercussions from poor results rather than just negligence put this union to the test. But it was managed care, especially under the rules of capitation that made this once-sacred relationship begin to falter. Under these restraints, physicians were now forced to recognize the needs of all patients within a particular funding system. No longer was it just about the one patient. Because of an expanding patient base, coupled with growing funding and resource limitations, physicians were incentivized to do less and sometimes penalized for doing more.

Along the way, the tide in physicians' attitudes also changed. No longer was medicine "their life." What was once a calling to most that had chosen the medical profession was becoming a vocation. Not because they were any less dedicated to their patients, but because the advances in technology not only within the medical profession, but also in the areas of telemedicine, cross-coverage, and communication, had freed them to devote more of their time to their families and other interests. The very technology that had brought health care to the highest level in the history of mankind was gradually stripping the emotion out of the relationship.

Instead of a stethoscope, an ophthalmoscope, and a reassuring pair of hands to probe for underlying pathology, many physicians of today turn to their monitors for answers. Have these advances raised the level of care? Unequivocally *yes*! If we ask if these advances have raised the level of caring, however, the answer is a resounding *no*!

A change in patients' expectations also plays a part. Increasingly, patients are basing their judgments on outcomes rather than efforts. Not that the trend is totally wrong, but in a science that is still in its infancy, much is still in transition. Patients did not come to feel this way on their own. Marketing of health care services has planted the seeds of unrealistic expectations. The media, in its attempt to inform, fails to paint the whole picture. Finally, the ravenous legal community stands by, threatening and watching to scoop up the remains from any adverse outcome.

Most of the rhetoric espoused during both the political conventions in the summer of 2012 followed traditional party lines. In his acceptance speech for the Republican Party's nomination for president, Governor Mitt Romney said that outside of one's chosen religious beliefs, the issues affecting the family unit were central to everything. This precept goes back to the basics of problem solving in mathematics—reduce the problem to its **lowest common denominator**. That similarity to our priorities in health care struck a note. Heath care reform, insurance coverage, preexisting conditions, liability concerns, fees, charges—the list goes on and on. Greater than all these elements, preserving the sanctity of the **doctor/patient relationship** must be central to everything debated in Washington, in the corridors of our hospitals, and in our offices. It doesn't matter whether the debate is about advances in the science, the fear of legal jeopardy, regulatory intervention, or who's paying the bill, that relationship must remain sacrosanct.

Not only do physicians put themselves in legal jeopardy, but they also incur scorn from the medical community when they abandon their patients. Abandonment doesn't always have to be just physical separation. Frequently overlooked are the deleterious effects when the loss of connection is emotional.

When patients refer to their doctors, but can't recall their names, or when doctors only remember their patients by their diagnoses, are examples of emotional abandonment by each party. Even more important, such physicians have failed to uphold the covenant our forefathers made with their patients many years ago.[3]

———

While most of medical education and training is about the nuts and bolts of clinical care—how to treat hypertension, how to manage a ventilator, how to take out a gallbladder—the process also involves learning how to be "a doctor." As opposed to lessons covered in textbooks and classrooms, this kind of learning is done through modeling, or what medical sociologist F. W. Hafferty has called the "informal" or "hidden curriculum."
—Tara Parker-Pope, New York Times, January 29, 2009

———

Etiquette-based communication employs five key strategies: introducing oneself, explaining one's role in the patient's care, touching the patient, asking open-ended questions such as "How are you feeling today" and sitting down with the patient.[3]

AXIOMS

1. Besides diagnosing and treating patients' maladies, the next priority is allaying their fears.

Even if the outcome does not appear to be favorable, the physician must try to allay the patients' fears. The most common fears are that they are facing the unknown, that they will be alone in their battle, and that they will suffer.

2. Establishing rapport is the first step that allows the physician to make the connection.

For the patient to "open up," the physician must divert the patient's concerns from just the malady—perhaps with an unrelated topic that interrupts the patient's fixation on his or her illness and gives the relationship another dimension. This can be a mutual interest—the football game on the television above the bed, for example. This allows the patient to sense the physician is interested in him or her and not just the diagnosis.

3. Patients need to feel they are getting their doctors' full attention during their encounter.

Some doctors always seem to be in a hurry. Often they have more pressing needs elsewhere. But for that brief moment, that particular patient should be the doctor's only concern. Comments like, "He always had his hand on the door" and "He looked like he was walking out, even when he was walking in," are often cited as examples. Any action or gesture that could be interpreted as preoccupation or showing a lack of concern must be avoided.

4. Doctors should try to direct their conversation to their patients, even when they may not be as able to understand as well as others who are with them.

Patients need to be part of the discourse at whatever level they are capable. Frequently cited examples are: "The doctor spent the whole time talking to his nurse. He never looked up from his chart. He never even looked at me." Finally often comes the plea, "I am perfectly capable of understanding." Even children after a certain age, the elderly, and the mentally challenged want to be part of the discourse if the problems concern them. Eye-to-eye contact often means as much as what is being said.

5. How much time should a physician spend with a patient? Patient encounters should not just be measured by allocated slots, only that there is "enough" time to listen to and address their concerns.

Even though the nurse or physician representative may have already taken a history, all patients need to "tell their story" to their doctor. Skill may be needed to direct the patient to recount only the cogent points. This is their initial investment in the relationship. Histories taken by others often do not convey the underlying concerns that can't be put down on paper. It is a transfer of the privately held concerns from the patient to *his or her* doctor.

6. For patients to be able to hear their doctors and really listen, physicians must first remove the barriers that block patients' ability to take in what they are being told.

Like the maestro of an orchestra, the physician must act as the facilitator, rather than dominate the encounter. Reading body language is essential. Looking at a relative, the nurse, or the chart can't do this. Examples such as "Everything is going to be OK" and "We will be able to handle your problem" often ameliorate some of their fears—those related to the fear of the unknown. The patients may not understand their problem, but now they know their doctor does or will find out.

7. Physicians should be sensitive when patients "open up" about a personal matter that may or may not pertain to their visit.

A "sensitive ear" may be one of the most effective therapies. It is important to remember that physicians are not just doctors of science, but doctors of patients with patience!

8. Never take away the patient's hope.

Even when the outlook is hopeless for a cure or a return to normalcy, the patient must not be left without hope. It is important that this is not false hope with unattainable expectations. The major fears of most patients with incurable conditions are being alone and suffering—a sense of hopelessness. These fears can be somewhat allayed by the physician, even when a cure is not likely.

9. Physicians should not come across as uncertain.

Even though the physician may be unsure of the correct cause and course of action, they he or she should not appear confused. "I don't know" with just a shrug, is totally different from "I don't know but…" followed by a plan that will help the patient in his or her quest for further understanding, comfort, guidance, and resolution.

10. Don't isolate patients by age or circumstances unless others are included.

Normal aging is progressive and not always a benign process. "You're just getting old" or "Your parts are wearing out." are troubling pronouncements when given in isolation. Much more acceptable would be, "We're all getting older." It softens the statement and puts one into a peer group with similar maladies.

11. The patient's concerns should never be trivialized.

"Minor surgery" is minor only after recovery! In the large scheme of things, a case of influenza in one patient is a lot less innocuous than acute lymphocytic leukemia in another, but not to each individual patient. The concerns of each patient are real to them and should never be trivialized. "I wouldn't worry about that," from a physician, can come across as showing a lack of concern, unless it is accompanied by some gesture of kindness.

12. Don't be critical of previous doctors.

Physicians frequently get into situations where they disagree either with the diagnosis or therapy of their patient by a previous physician. It is difficult to not be critical. Unless the previous care is egregious, it is best to avoid any criticism for several reasons:

a) Patients still have some carryover loyalty to their previous physician.
b) The new physician must establish trust with the new patient. Questioning the actions of the previous doctor can often raise concerns about the current physician too.
c) The current physician could be wrong.

Phrases like "I wasn't there when your problems first arose" or "Doctors often have different approaches" tend to negate patients' concerns if there is disagreement among physicians. At the same time, the current physician can use the patient's trust in the previous physician to build rapport in this "new" relationship.

13. Patients should be informed about their problems to the extent that it is in their best interest.

The unknown only breeds more fear. Patients can imagine anything, and frequently it is the worst. Even when it hurts, the truth is always the best option. However, when the patient is unable to understand or cope with reality, unexaggerated reassurance is suggested, and the physician should fully inform the patient's next of kin or legal proxy.

14. Patients should always be made to feel that they are a part of the decision making when it comes to their own care.

By its very nature, there is an imbalance of power in the patient/doctor relationship. As long as the outcomes are not compromised, and there are alternatives, patients should always feel involved in making decisions that affect them.

15. Physicians should not contradict themselves.

Although patients usually don't remember everything their physician tells them, they are, at the least, attentive to every word the physician tells them. Changing the message without an explanation only leads to confusion. Mundane as it sounds, asking a patient to return in two weeks, then changing it to three weeks, often creates a great deal of concern.

16. Allow the patient an opportunity for questions at the end of the visit.

Don't leave the encounter without an attempt at closure. This final gesture is a way to see if the patient has a grasp on the situation. Even then there are times the patient doesn't "hear" what he or she has been told because of the stress and preoccupation of the situation.

—

We would like doctors to listen, but the fact is, we better be ready to be able to talk to them. You're going to have to be an active participant in that conversation, so I'd say the American people are going to need ways of stepping up to the conversation.
—Anna Deavere Smith, American actress

Societal changes have altered the once hallowed patient/doctor relationship. The introduction of third-party payers has probably had the most effect. No longer is it just the patient who is responsible for the costs of his or her care. Now the third parties become the intermediary. Patients develop an entitlement mind-set. They paid their premiums, and now they are "owed" their care. No longer do they serve as their own gatekeepers, whether it is determining when to seek medical advice or seeking exposure to any and all diagnostics and therapeutics available. The responsibility for balance between costs and needs has been taken over by their intermediary. This shift to the third-party payer potentially makes the patient/doctor relationship more adversarial for both the patients and their physicians.

17. Doctors must strive to be intermediaries between their patients and the third-party payers.

Despite the rules set down by the third-party payers, physicians must always act as advocates for their patients.

18. Loyalty to the patient's best interest must take precedence over loyalty to the third-party payer.

Although physicians have a divided responsibility to maintain the viability of the third-party payers to ensure reasonable access for other patients within the payment plan, their first loyalty is to that one patient.

19. Physicians should make their patients aware of all diagnostic studies and therapies that could help them.

Even though these resources may not be available or affordable, patients deserve that awareness. No longer is medicine practiced in isolation. If there are new or more advanced therapies or laboratory tests, patients will eventually hear about them. This type of information is always better coming from their doctor.

In the event a patient chooses to pursue other options, the physician should assist the patient in that pursuit, even if it is outside their area or payment system. This might only involve making them aware of the other choices or, in some cases, playing a more active role. However, these obligations don't apply if the physician feels these options are not in the patient's best interest.

There has been a change in patients' acceptance of undesirable outcomes. What may have once been considered an "act of God" is now often attributed to negligence. Anytime a procedure or therapy does not fulfill patients' expectations, questions are raised. Now the first thing that comes to mind is blame[5]—not a fault in an understanding of the science (an "act of God" concept), but rather a fault by the provider. If there is blamable injury, then restitution becomes a reasonable expectation for patients. When that tension occurs, patients sometimes contact an attorney while physicians put in a call to their malpractice insurance carrier. Again the patient/physician relationship becomes critically disrupted.

Why the change? Three major factors: (1) marketing by the providers of health care services that almost guarantees results; (2) the mass media, which does not paint the whole picture; and (3) the legal community, which confuses poor outcomes with negligence. Each of these entities distorts the patients' expectations and often raises them to unrealistic levels.

Doctors are men who prescribe medicines of which they know little, to cure diseases of which they know less, in human beings of whom they know nothing.
—*Voltaire, French writer and historian, 1694–1778*

20. **Physicians should not promise results based on outcomes, only for their services.**

It is often forgotten that although the practice of medicine has become "big business," it is still a science in its infancy and therefore fraught with unpredictable outcomes. More money does not always buy better results.

21. Physicians should guarantee efforts but not outcomes.

Marketing influences patient selection into the science of medicine. With advances, the predictability of outcomes increases, but never to 100 percent.

Outcomes are often predictable but never certain. Less than ideal results of a therapy or a surgery are better accepted if patients have realistic expectations. Marketing promises often create false expectations.

22. Physicians should not become upset or feel threatened if patients question their recommendations.

Patients may no longer accept as absolute what their physicians tell them. The mass media has not only raised patients' expectations; it has also raised their doubts. Patients have the right to question or even ask for a second opinion. Physicians have a responsibility to listen to their patients and help them work through their concerns.

23. Physicians should confine their practices to their area of expertise.

The growth in the medical sciences allows physicians to expand their skill sets. Concurrently, this must be accompanied with the proper training and background. Often physicians and "substitute" doctors branch off into new areas. Even though their training in this new direction may appear adequate, if the foundation of prior knowledge and expertise is not there, problems may occur.

24. Physicians should never prescribe a therapy or perform a procedure if they either are unable to handle the complications or cannot readily transfer the patient to someone who can.

The "best" physicians know what they do not know and whom to consult.

25. Medical errors must be dealt with openly and honestly.

Diagnostic and therapeutic errors are an unfortunate consequence of human fallibility and the unpredictability of the science of medicine. Experience and attention to detail make these errors more predictable and often preventable. Since errors occur in all human interactions, their recognition, correction, explanation, regret, and apology should be promptly forthcoming. A patient (or family) is likely to be more understanding when the discussion occurs in close proximity to the event and, when indicated, consultation is recommended.[4,5]

26. The best way avoid a lawsuit is to tell the truth.

The "art" of medicine is all about communication with the patient. By explaining up front the real risks and likelihood of outcomes and by being error conscious, the physician is more apt to avoid undesirable outcomes. Even if the results turn out not as hoped for, then at least they were not unexpected. Dialogue trumps an operation permit every time.

27. In the face of adversity, it is even more important for the physician to be supportive and communicative.

When the course of a patient's recovery is not going as hoped, physicians should step in and be supportive. With growing uncertainty, far too often physicians shy away from confrontations. Like patients and loved ones, physicians are also uncomfortable. This is not the time for resentment, anger, or making excuses. Being communicative and directly confronting the difficulties head on bring stability back to the relationship.

28. Like children, patients need boundaries.

It is vital that patients comply with their physicians' recommendations. Failure to comply potentially hurts the patient. Although physicians can't force compliance, if necessary, they can refuse to continue to care for these patients. Doctors have an obligation to offer their patients appropriate care. Sometimes it is necessary to utilize "tough love" by forcing patients to seek that care elsewhere by facilitating a transfer of responsibility.

29. Physicians must not confuse their role as a doctor with that of a friend or family member.

Although friendship brings trust to a relationship, it also threatens objectivity. If there must be a choice, then the role as a physician takes precedent. Examples are parents who also try to be their children's best friend or physicians who treat their close family members for a serious illness or injury.

30. Showing appreciation helps patients develop more of a sense of "ownership" and trust in their physician.

In most situations patients have, at least, some choice in the selection of their physicians. Emergencies and managed care are often exceptions. Even without a prior relationship, physicians should appreciate and can build on the trust that patients hold for anyone who is a physician. Part of establishing rapport with patients is the "human" trait of humility.

31. Physicians must not abandon their patients.

If a physician feels that he or she cannot continue a relationship with a particular patient for any reason, then that physician should make arrangements to transfer the patient to another qualified caregiver. During the time the transfer is taking place, the physician is still responsible for any emergencies until the transfer is completed.

32. Physicians should not be afraid to touch their patients.

In a day when almost any advance can be construed as inappropriate, physicians must not be forced to abandon actions that ensure commitment. A gentle touch, a reassuring smile, and eye contact are sometimes the most effective therapy during difficult situations. At the very least, they are gestures of kindness and connection.

33. Kindness might just be the best treatment physicians can give their patients.[5,6]

———

Is it not also true that no physician, in so far as he is a physician, considers or enjoins what is for the physician's interest, but that all seek the good of their patients? For we have agreed that a physician strictly so called, is a ruler of bodies, and not a maker of money, have we not?

—Plato, Greek philosopher, 427–347 BC

2.

Interactions with Fellow Physicians and Health Care Workers

There are various situations where physicians interact with other physicians and other practitioners—physician assistants, nurse practitioners, chiropractors, just to name a few. These interactions serve to transfer information intended to benefit the care of patients and disperse knowledge among those who care for them. For these relationships to be fruitful, certain standards of conduct should be followed.

There are courtesies that physicians or their representatives who request consultations and the physicians who answer them should follow. The requesting parties are asking the consultants to interrupt their normal schedule to see patients, while the parties being consulted are being complimented for their expertise.

AXIOMS

For physicians starting their practices:

1. Introduce yourself to the physicians to whom you hope to refer patients and to consult.

Although there are several approaches, such as announcement cards, newspaper announcements, and visitation, the latter is the most productive.

2. **Marketing one's practice sets the tone to the physician community as to how the entering physician (or even an established physician) intends to conduct his or her practice.**

Until relatively recently, marketing, which is a more professional term for advertising, was generally frowned upon. Traditionally, the physician community relied on "word of mouth" and the methods described in axiom 1 to announce and grow their practices.

Although marketing practices are now legal, they potentially raise concerns about an individual physician's priorities. These practices may also affect the standing of physicians who advertise within the community as well as the physicians who do not.

For physicians requesting consultations:

3. **Attempt to contact the consulting physician directly.**

Physicians should be sensitive that the request may cause an inconvenience for the consulting physician. The direct contact also is more likely to convey pertinent information about the patient's history and specific questions. This is much preferred to simply writing an order on the patient's chart or having a nurse or a physician's assistant place the call. It also demonstrates respect when physicians initiate the contact personally.

4. **When requesting the consultation, do not make the consultant wait.**

Although emergent situations can be the exception, being called to the telephone only to be told to wait while the person on the other end of the line gets the physician is aggravating. Remember, the party who initiated the call is the one making the request.

5. **Always express appreciation to the consulting physician.**

Physicians who are asked to assist in the diagnosis and treatment of a patient are not only providing a service, they are doing the requesting physician a favor.

For physicians responding to consultations:

6. Never criticize the care of the referring physician or another practitioner.

If there is a problem that can't be easily rectified, then the requesting physician should be contacted. If the problem is egregious, then the proper authorities should be notified. In virtually every case of this nature, except in emergencies, the patient should only be made aware of the situation after the requesting physician or the proper authorities have been notified.

7. If the consulting physician feels additional expertise is necessary, the requesting physician should be notified first.

This is a courtesy owed the originating physician to not "leave them out of the loop." He or she is still the patient's primary doctor and should be recognized as such. The exceptions are emergent and urgent situations where multiple disciplines may be necessary.

8. Being consulted is a compliment.

Physicians should recognize that, when asked to consult, they are being honored. With that request comes a responsibility for the well-being of their new patient, but also the responsibility to preserve the existing patient/doctor relationship when their role is finished. Otherwise, the next time, their expertise may not be requested.

9. Always report back to the consulting physician or practitioner.

There are several methods available: writing in the progress notes of the patients' charts, telephones calls, pre-stamped cards with blank spaces to fill in, texts, e-mails, or letters. Although different encounters call for varying responses, the more personal the response, the better.

Do not underestimate the importance of physicians' relations with others in health care delivery. The practice of medicine is not just rendering care. It is orchestrating the laboratory results, the radiological findings, and pathology reports with colleagues and a number of various disciplines.

10. There is no excuse for being rude.

Whether it is a nurse, a medical assistant, a technician, or one of the numerous professionals in a variety of medical disciplines who call themselves doctors, there is no excuse for being rude. Although, as physicians, we may not always agree with another's approach, we share the same goals—helping patients. Without the assistance of other medical practitioners, physicians often cannot carry out their roles.

11. No one physician or practitioner has all the answers.

It is important to remember that the basic tenets upon which allopathic medicine was founded are carried with us throughout our practice lives. Variations from those founding principles are sometimes interpreted as without value. The future evolution of the science will prove the validity or lack of validity of these other disciplines. If allowing these alternative approaches to health care delivery is felt to be harmful, physicians should make their patients aware of their concerns.

12. Honoring "professional courtesy" does not always follow strict guidelines.

Traditionally, physicians have not charged their fellow physicians, their spouses, their dependent children, and sometimes members of the clergy, beyond "insurance only" benefits.

Elective plastic surgery and psychiatry are two specialties where this is not routinely followed. The reasons given are that the surgery is cosmetic and not essential or, in psychiatry, that it is an integral part of the therapy and gives the patients a sense of ownership in their recovery. Often included in these restrictions are elective appliances, such as contact lenses.

Questions arise when the physician dies and the spouse lives on, when there is a divorce, or when the child has "grown up" but still is financially dependent on the family. These situations must be handled on an individual basis.

13. Physicians serve as role models for other physicians and future physicians.

The image usually begins long before medical school:

"The physician that cared for them when they were younger. The physician, who tried to save their mother, but comforted them when her heart finally gave out. The physician who performed the first heart transplant."[7]

These have been medicine's traditional role models. Today, that face is changing—for example, the photo of the physician in his freshly pressed suit and perfectly folded handkerchief that adorns the center of a page in an airline magazine is an example of commercialism that is gradually changing the physicians' image. Many physicians see these opposing images and question that they want to emulate.

14. Physicians have an obligation to police the medical profession.

Acts of fraud by members of the medical community are being reported with increasing frequency. It is debatable whether they are on the increase or whether the ability to discover them has improved. These occurrences cast aspersions throughout a profession that relies on trust as an integral part of its ability to care for the sick and injured. Awareness of fraud, without acting to report or rectify it, could be considered as complicit as committing the fraudulent act itself.[2]

3.

Interactions with Hospital Representatives

The relationship between physicians and hospitals is one of codependency. Each party needs the trust of the other. The reason is often money and reputation. In some ways this love/hate relationship occurred before the third-party payers and federal funding programs stepped in. Physicians needed a place to care for their sickest patients, and hospitals needed to fill their beds. In those earlier days, many hospitals had some support from charitable organizations. By and large, the costs of delivery were lower, so much of the losses were written off without much financial peril to the institutions. Even today, a few of these institutions still get supplements. Most of that changed when medicine became a big business controlled by federal guidelines and third-party payer reimbursements. Even the so-called charity institutions are subject to these same constraints.

Physicians are caught between the best interests of their patients and the tight-fisted oversight adopted by the hospitals. Length of hospital stays, complication rates, and percentage of readmissions are related in part to the bottom line. Reimbursement rates have become the primary hospital concern. Hospitals are forced to offer an array of services that are not profitable in order to stay competitive. Many less serious procedures and diagnostics that are the most profitable have been moved out of the hospitals and into privately owned, for-profit centers.

With increasing profits in the private centers and growing constraints on the traditional hospitals, physician loyalty to hospitals has been diminishing. Trying to stay afloat, hospitals began employing physicians and buying up the practices of others. In other cases, hospitals began building and buying up profit centers and encouraging physicians to invest in them. These new alliances have created sharp divides within the physician community—between those physicians who have potential conflicts of interest because they are financially linked to the hospitals and those who remain independent.

In both situations, the basic interactions among physicians should not change. However, the relations among the physicians who are employed or vested with the hospitals and those who remain independent take on a whole new perspective. The former now have two roles: advocates for their patients and partners with the hospitals.

AXIOMS

For physicians employed or vested by hospitals:

1. Physicians' primary concerns must still be in the best interests of their patients.

Physicians cannot abrogate patient responsibility even if it puts them in conflict with the hospital.

2. Physicians are advocates for all the patients undergoing treatment in their facility.

Physicians must work to ensure that the quality of care in *their* institution or facility is not compromised for any reason.

3. Physicians must work to ensure the continuing viability of their institution.

As vested partners or employees, physicians are bound to utilize the assets of their hospitals in the most efficient and prudent manner. Without this sense of awareness and obligation, the institution will not prosper, and the patients may suffer!

4. Since physicians are in partnership with the representatives of the hospital, they should treat them in a collegial manner.

These physicians are now in the "business of medicine" and must act accordingly to their associates. However, they must never lose sight that the needs of their patients must always come first.

For independent physicians:

5. Physicians must advocate for maintaining the best diagnostics and therapeutics available in the facility where they admit their patients.

Physicians' loyalty to their patients is paramount to their loyalty to the institution.

6. Physicians should strive to support improved services at the hospitals, ancillary facilities, laboratories, and extended care institutions where they care for patients. If that cannot be accomplished, they should attempt to transfer their patients' care elsewhere.

4.

Interactions with Pharmaceutical and Medical Device Companies

Dear Doctor: *May 1935*

Together with congratulations on your attainment of a medical degree, this volume of addresses by Sir William Osler who adorned your profession in the United States for so many years is cordially presented.

As the addresses by this master-mind of modern medicine are read, may you catch his vision of the almost boundless possibilities of your chosen profession.

May you share with him his "relish of knowledge" and his absorbing love and passionate, persistent search for truth.

Above all, may there come to you an inspiration which will enable you to live a rich, a happy and abundant life.

Sincerely yours,
Eli Lilly
President: Eli Lilly and Company[8]

Pharmaceutical and medical device companies function between two potentially conflicting agendas: profit and the beneficence of the relief of suffering. Physicians must sort through these somewhat opposing goals so as to benefit their patients' best interests. Even though these companies' products have been invaluable in bringing the level of medical care to where it is today, these institutions are still businesses and incorporate business practices in order to sell their products. To perpetuate their company, the "bottom line" is one measure of their success.

Without profits they cannot continue their research and development. They survive by an influx of funds from sales, grants, and investors who expect a return on their investment. Physicians must appreciate this equation called capitalism, which improves the quality of care while at the same time creates a profit for stockholders and advances the long-term goals of their company.

AXIOMS

1. Pharmaceutical and medical device company representatives should be complimentary to physicians' practices.

They play a valuable role in two ways: First is physician education about the merits of their latest products over existing modalities and those of their competition. Second is a source of the product sampled so physicians can gain experience with its use and provide it for needy patients. To ignore these representatives and their message only denies physicians a valuable source of information and their patients' access to the latest medications. It is the responsibility of the physicians to act as evaluators of new products based on effectiveness, margin of safety, convenience of administration, and cost.

2. Physicians should be aware of potential conflicts of interest in personal relationships with pharmaceutical representatives.

Pharmaceutical representatives are the messengers. Their job is to promote their company's products, and their success is measured by how many prescriptions are written or devices ordered by the physicians they call upon. Their primary purpose is to put their company's products in the best light.

3. Physicians should not accept gifts or benefits of significant value that would influence their prescribing patterns.

Samples and seminars should have only two effects: physician education and patient benefit. Even though the pharmaceutical and medical device companies have begun to establish standards for their industry, physicians must not let themselves be unduly influenced by their promotional activities.

4. Physicians should not require benefits from pharmaceutical company representatives in order to allow access.

The prerequisite of a free lunch for the physician and the office staff diminishes the dignity of the profession. Physicians should not be "bought" even if the purchase is considered a pittance. However, if the representative's visit interrupts or delays the physician's schedule, then providing modest nourishment seems appropriate.

5. If physicians obtain remuneration from a pharmaceutical or medical device company for recommendations or services, full disclosure of that relationship must be clearly made known to any and all potential audiences and patients.

Physicians are a valuable resource for these companies, both in the initial research and the encouragement of others to use their products once on the market. Whether it is by presentations and seminars or through publications, full disclosure of any potential conflict of interest must be made known.

5.

Interactions with Third-Party Payers

Blue Cross/Blue Shield first began providing health care coverage in 1929. President Lyndon Johnson signed the Social Security Amendments of 1965 into law, which was the genesis of the Medicaid and Medicare programs. But it wasn't until the 1980s that these payers of health care service begin to significantly exert their influence into the practice of medicine. From that point on, there has been a torrent of regulations and restrictions that not only tell physicians what they will be reimbursed, but also what they can charge, how long treatments should take, and even what diagnostics and therapeutics they should use. The latest in this litany of rulings is reimbursing physicians based on outcomes.

AXIOMS

1. There is no going back to the way it was before.

Delivery of health care services is big business. An enlarging patient population, a more demanding public, and an explosion in technological advances have moved medicine past the point when costs were not a determining factor in the larger equation of health care delivery.

2. Patients should be informed of all medical charges in advance, with the exception of emergency services.

There is no other current commodity or service where the purchaser or the provider of the service does not know the charges in advance of the service being rendered!

3. Third-party payers are unavoidable.

We no longer function in an age where most health care, when available, was an act of beneficence. In a civilized society, patients should be guaranteed a basic level of health care services. For those who don't have the funds to cover their services, some form of supplementation must be available. In this country this is through emergency rooms, charity clinics, or some form of federal funding mechanism (i.e., Medicaid, etc.). Even these entities that furnish free services must get their funding from some source. These expenses are too high to be written off, and, except in rare circumstances, charitable contributions are not sufficient to fill these needs.

4. Physicians should act as intermediaries between their patients and the third-party payers when necessary.

Although patients choose their own coverage, they are subject to the dictums of their third-party provider. They have a responsibility for their own expenses but often are not "informed" with respect to their benefits. Most often they don't read or even understand the provisions outlined in the "fine print" of their policies. Physicians and their staff do.

Physicians who abrogate this role not only leave their patients at the mercy of the payer, but they potentially hinder their own reimbursement.

5. Physicians should make their patients aware of the coverage limits and benefits of their health care policies.

Patients are often naive about what services their coverage provides and what it does not. Unless the service is considered urgent, and delay could potentially cause harm, physicians should inform patients about the costs of any services not covered under their policy. In an urgent situation, the patient's need must be served, preceding his or her ability to pay.

6. If reimbursement levels are too low for a particular service, physicians should work with the payer to bring them up to appropriate levels.

This action to deal with appropriate fee schedules might be on a case-by-case basis. On a broader basis, physicians are much more effective agents of change if they join with other physicians or organizations that represent them.

7. Physicians should encourage patients not to abrogate their responsibility with their own health care carrier.

Patients often feel "entitled" when it comes to the responsibility for their own bill once they have purchased coverage. They feel it is up to their doctor to "work it out" with the insurer. Shifting this responsibility completely to the doctor potentially harms the patient/doctor relationship. Even with coverage, patients still bear a responsibility to ensure their provider is fulfilling their obligations.

8. Physicians have a responsibility to ensure that the charges for their services have been submitted in a timely and appropriate manner to the third-party payers.

Although the statements may be submitted by patients or directly to the payer, physicians have a responsibility to ensure that the appropriate coding and diagnoses are utilized.

9. If a physician suspects that health care fraud has taken place, he or she has a moral and legal obligation to bring it to the attention of the proper authorities.

The medical profession was built on a foundation of trust and honesty. Turning a blind eye not only perpetuates a system of deceit, but it allows large sums of money to be diverted away from more appropriate services. Abdication of these obligations necessitates more government intervention into the practice of medicine.

6.

Interactions with the Public's Elected Representatives

Physicians play three roles when interacting with their elected representatives: as individual voters, as advocates for patients, and as representatives of the medical profession. In most situations, the position of an individual physician as related to a particular issue will be the same for all three roles. But this is not always the case.

As voters, physicians have the right to shed their role as doctors and vote for individuals who best support issues that affect them and their families personally and society at large. Similarly, physicians have a responsibility to support elected individuals who represent what is best for their patients and an improved community. Even then, there can be conflicts if an issue can affect the whole of the medical profession. The question arises, if there is a conflict, of which role takes precedent.

AXIOMS

1. If physicians want to address issues that affect them, their families, their patients, or the medical profession, they must become involved.

Conflicts are not won "sitting on the sidelines." The ability to give meaningful input is best accomplished by making connections with elected representatives. Giving support to others or organizations that embrace similar interests also adds to this effectiveness.

2. "All politics is local."

This often-quoted axiom points out that one vote from a constituent is more important than a dollar from a donor. Although elected representatives rely on funds and volunteers to support their elections, the one thing that puts them and keeps them in office is the vote by their constituents. Professional action committees and special interests groups have influence, but not as much as the voters.

Physicians can make a difference with their donations and by joining with organizations that support their interests. However, the real influence comes from their personal relationships with the candidates and by working (spouses and family members included) in their campaigns.

3. Being right is not always enough.

Until relatively recently, physicians have assumed that if they stood by their principles involving health care, any issues would be resolved in their favor. That myth evaporated with the expansion of medical privileges by non-physicians though the state legislatures.

It's a political world. Like it or not, physicians must join the process, or they will be left behind.

4. Physicians will never get ahead if they are always reactive and not proactive.

If physicians just wait around to defend themselves against the next onslaught of regulations and intrusions, they will never move forward. Health care reform legislation is a perfect example. This involves campaigning on two fronts: putting up a good defense, but also laying out legislation that will address the concerns and, then electing and/or finding support to get those proposals enacted.

5. Those who are for or against any issue are the most effective when their opposition can be fractionated.

Most elected representatives are more concerned about final solutions to legislative issues than how those solutions are derived. Thus, if differing physician groups present different solutions, the elected representative will usually rule in favor of the most politically expedient solution. The differing interests within the physician community should be addressed within the organizations that represent them rather than in the halls of Congress or the state legislatures.

6. On issues that affect patients, physicians' input within the political process is invaluable.

Physicians should not shy away from educating their patients about issues that affect their care. This must be in a time-appropriate manner and not take away from the importance of the patient's visit.

7. Compromise in politics is inevitable.

The definition of politics almost always infers compromise. The term politics is used to describe the interactions of dealing with differing interests. If one party had their way all the time, there would be no need for interaction...thus, no politics.

Physicians find this process especially difficult because of the noble cause they serve. Anything less than their goal usually means their patients get less of whatever the competing issue involves.

The success in this process is to be able to discern which points can be compromised and which cannot.

8. Since almost 80 percent of health care spending is directed by physicians, they should take more of a leadership position

regarding rules that are made and how health care funds are allocated.

If physicians don't involve themselves in the political process, they cannot expect to have significant influence in determining the outcomes. They have a responsibility to weigh the value of the costs generated by the diagnostics they order and the treatments they prescribe.

———

I'm strongly for a patient Bill of Rights. Decisions ought to be made by doctors, not accountants.
—Charles Schumer, United States senator

7.

Interactions with State and Federal Regulators

Although the states have exercised some control over the practice of medicine for a long time, their jurisdiction was more control over physician behavior through licensure. It wasn't until the creation of the federal subsidy programs, Medicare and Medicaid, in 1965 that federal guidelines began to affect the way health care was delivered. In the 1970s, the intrusions started out with fairly innocuous payment limits to patients for their treatments. Over the last quarter of the twentieth century, that trickle of changes has turned into a deluge of regulations that now permeate every level of the care delivery system in this country.

The ever-growing patient population, the exploding array of diagnostics and therapeutics, and the escalating costs for patient care are on a collision course. There is no end in sight.

Interactions between the providers of health care services and the agencies and individuals who are responsible for regulating and funding the resources are strained at best.

AXIOMS

1. In many situations the regulators are just the messengers.

Enforcing compliance with laws passed by our elected representatives is usually the reason for regulations. Often the laws establish an agency that is necessary to ensure compliance with the law.

These agencies then issue regulations to ensure the dictums of the law are carried out.

Although there are mechanisms to contest these rules and regulations when they are first promulgated, the appeals process is very time sensitive and usually cumbersome. Those who protest must usually resort to the courts, which are slow and expensive, or readdress the problems through the legislative pathway.

2. The regulators are not physicians' friends, but they are not the enemy either.

The regulators' job, like that of IRS agents, is to ensure compliance. If they only utilize punitive measures, it not only creates discord, but also fosters an atmosphere of noncompliance.

3. Physicians should stand their ground if they feel the regulations infringe on their ability to care for their patients or compromise the extent and quality of their care.

Physicians may voice their objectives to regulations with which they disagree. They have an obligation to try to address any wrongs that are being done to them or their patients. This may be by their efforts or through organizations that represent physicians. Doing nothing in the face of injustices only encourages further intrusions into the practice of medicine.

4. Physicians must not participate with their patients in extorting the funding system.

Patients often feel they are being treated unfairly by the payment system. A frequent recourse by them is to try to "bend the rules," and they often want their physician to go along. Besides being illegal, there are several things wrong with this. First, if discovered, not only is the doctor in jeopardy, but the patient is put in jeopardy too. Most important, the physician should not compromise his or her integrity.

8.

Interactions with Medical, Dental, and Public Health Organizations

Nonparticipation is a growing epidemic in this country. It crosses all levels of society and many of the traditional organizations, including those that represent physicians.

The problem with decreased participation can be diminished goals and, in the case of medical organizations, the potential loss of influence in political arenas. As new physicians enter medicine, there appears be less concern about matters that affect the whole of the profession and more about their own area of interest. Thus, those with the authority (elected leaders) to make decisions that affect medicine are often being approached with differing messages that allow them more control over the profession. With the growing number of "employed" physicians, there is increasing concern that *medicine's voice* will even become more divided, more distant, and less effective.

AXIOMS

1. Physicians bear a responsibility to advocate for what is in the best interests of their patients.

Physicians owe their patients more than just providing them the best medical care available. They have a responsibility to act as advocates between their patients and those entities that might deprive them of the care and preventive health services to which they are entitled.

2. Physicians bear a responsibility to their community and the whole of the medical profession.

Although it may not always be obvious, physicians do not practice in isolation. The very knowledge they were taught in the early part of their training was a gift from many patients and physicians who came before them. The freedoms they exercise are because others championed to preserve them. Upon entering the profession, all physicians assume responsibilities to not only work to preserve what they enjoy, but to work to advance and grow the community for future generations of physicians and their patients.

3. Physicians should support organizations that represent the medical profession's best interests and those of their patients.

Support by physicians does not have to be active participation. It could be in dues dollars only. However, making these organizations more effective would involve physicians giving input on critical issues to make them more representative and less autocratic of their membership.

4. Physicians should not abandon organizations that disagree with them on certain issues if those positions have been decided by a democratic process.

Democratically run organizations will most often differ with at least one participant on almost every issue. Rarely does complete unanimity exist. It becomes important that the factions accept their differences and don't quit because they don't always agree. Some party is going to be asked to make decisions on difficult issues. These decisions should be made by those who are the best informed.

5. Organizations that claim to represent physicians must be open to reflecting the changes in their members' needs and ideals.

One priority of medical organizations is to protect their members from change that would negatively affect their ability to practice medicine as they deem appropriate. Of almost equal importance is to be able to make changes in their own structure and governance that reflect the desires and needs of their physician members.

9.

Interactions with the Media

In the last two decades of the twentieth century and the dawning of the twenty-first century, changes in media culture and influence have permeated virtually every aspect of today's society. Internet, radio, television, and print media are now an integral part of the social fabric. What used to be just news and entertainment has transformed into a vehicle that influences almost every decision the public makes.

News is no longer just news. What the public hears and sees is now filtered. The truth is not necessarily the truth, just what the originator of the information wants the truth to be. *Propaganda* is a term coined to refer to information meant to influence. Any truths are of secondary importance. The more astute realize that the source of the information is as important as the facts, which are molded and packaged to fit the source's particular point of view.

Many in the medical profession have adopted these techniques as methods to expand their sphere of influence. What was considered a violation of ethical standards (advertising) fifty years ago is now the norm (marketing).

According to most state medical licensing boards and the American Medical Association, there are no restrictions on advertising by physicians except those that can be specifically justified to protect the public from deceptive practices.[2]

The consequence of this evolution is a better informed, but more doubting, public. In medicine, marketing techniques move the interactions between the physicians and their patients from relational to transactional, and from results based on efforts to outcomes.

AXIOMS

1. Physicians should not allow the media to use their name and reputation to manipulate the truth.

In an attempt to establish credibility, the media often incorporates testimony from medical experts. It is a use of the physician's reputation to enhance the media representative's credibility. This inclusion can be valuable as long as the message is correct and not intended to unduly influence a particular perspective.

2. It is important be able to differentiate informational from marketing pieces.

Far too often, information that would appear to educate turns out to be a pulpit for physicians and health care institutions to "market" their services. Sometimes they are able to accomplish both. Clear boundaries should be drawn as to the relationship between the author of a particular piece and the "medical experts" whose expertise is being included.

3. Marketing by physicians or health care institutions through the media should be labeled as such.

It should be reasonable to assume that if profit motive was not the primary intent of a particular piece, then those same monies could reach more patients through entities that speak for a larger segment of the health care community. As an example, money spent by an institution discussing the latest techniques in a particular cardiac service could arguably be better spent if donated to a national cardiology organization to deliver a similar message.

4. Although it appears to be an honor to be included in "Best Doctor" lists, the purpose of the publisher is to sell more advertising space and more magazines or papers.

"Best Doctor" lists are flawed from the start. First, the publisher's primary incentive is monetary and not public good. Second, they are wringing money out of the health care dollar by coaxing physicians to buy advertising space under the guise of providing information about doctors. Third, they are more often popularity contests than true evaluations of physician competence. Finally, they potentially create doubts in the minds of patients whose physicians are not included on the list.

10.

Interactions with the Public

When physicians communicate with the public, it can be through several different venues and to two potentially different audiences. The venues could be through the recognized media (periodicals, Internet, radio, or television) or personal encounters. The audiences can be separated into patients or potential patients and those who might never be patients. There should be a clear distinction in any of these interactions as to whether the physician is speaking as an individual or on behalf of the profession.

AXIOMS

When physicians speak for themselves:

1. As long as their remarks are not false or misleading, physicians can extol their own skills and attributes.

Physicians have the right—and, some would claim, the obligation—to make the public aware of their particular skill sets. Without this knowledge, patients are disadvantaged in making decisions about the selection of a health care provider.

Although naming names creates some legal jeopardy, physicians can compare their abilities to others who claim to have the same level of training and experience. This is especially important in comparison with non-physician practitioners.

2. Physicians should refrain from putting out information until it has passed the scrutiny of the scientific community.

Those within the medical profession have an obligation to share new discoveries and scientific advances quickly with the rest of the community (medical and nonmedical). There is also a counter-obligation to ensure this information has been properly researched before dissemination.

3. Physicians have the right to express their own political and religious beliefs as long as this doesn't put undue pressure on any current patient/doctor relationships with which they are involved.

Just because physicians have vowed to uphold the best interests of their patients does not imply they must abandon their own personal beliefs. However, physicians hold an unequal balance of power with their own patients that should not be used to achieve goals that are beyond the normal influence derived from their care.

When physicians speak for the profession:

4. All physicians represent the profession.

Once the MD is attached to their name, individuals can never really separate themselves from the medical profession. Even if their state license has been revoked or they are imprisoned for a heinous crime, they are still doctors of medicine. It is the first thing that catches one's eye in a news story or an obituary. Just as an elephant will always be an elephant, whatever any physician does is construed by some as a reflection of the medical profession.

5. If physicians serve as spokespeople for a medical organization or group, they must publically disclose support for the policies of that organization.

Although they may not personally agree with a particular position, that difference should only be made known to others within the organization they represent.

6. Physicians who serve as spokespeople for an organization or group should not make policy.

A spokesperson for a medical organization or group cannot create policy that is different from the dictums of the organization they represent. If any physician disagrees with the positions held by the group they represent, they should work to change those positions within the policy-making process of the group.

11.

Interactions with Oneself and the Family

Reflecting as to why they first chose medicine as a career, doctors come up with several recurring answers: They want to help others. They want a career that ensures them both job and financial security. They were science majors in college, and medicine seemed like their best option. One answer that does not come up often was that they wanted to make a lot of money.

Most knew the requirements going in: above average intelligence, dedication, sacrifice, and hard work. In the end, those who made the eight- to ten-year commitment after college could call themselves doctors of medicine. Their choices didn't end there. Even though most went into direct patient care, many dedicated doctors chose teaching, research, administration, and consulting positions. If they stayed in the field of medicine, they virtually all shared one thing in common—what they did, directly or indirectly, benefited people.

At some point in physicians' careers, there comes a time when the priorities that first led them into medicine have to be reevaluated. For some, the suffering of their patients had made them even more committed to their cause. For others, the years of sacrifice, doing without, and the multitude of constraints heaped on their ability to apply their talents have changed their priorities from results to rewards.

Whatever their status, they are torn between fulfillment and frustration. Although their patients are still their concern, patients are not and should not be their *only* concern.

Three of my children are medical doctors, they know at least a hundred times as much about your body as my grandfather knew, but they don't know much more about soul than he did.
—John Templeton, investor and mutual fund pioneer, 1912–2008

AXIOMS

When relating to physicians' own needs and those of their family:

1. The physician's own heath care needs must be a top priority.

If physicians don't attend to their own physical and mental health, they are also potentially abrogating their responsibilities to their patients, their families, and their employees. Being self-neglectful potentially compromises their judgment and impedes continued learning, future earnings, and the ability to continue to care for their patients and support their families.

2. Physicians must continue to learn and keep abreast of the latest and best diagnostic and therapeutic options in their area of area of expertise.

It has been said that without continuing education physicians are "out-of-date" every seven years. The science of medicine continues to expand at an exponential rate—thus, the reason for specialization and sub-specialization. Physicians have an obligation to their patients and themselves to remain informed.

3. Physicians must never lose their objectivity.

Whether it is pertaining to their patients, their families, or themselves, physicians must not let emotion cloud their judgment as to the best course of therapy to pursue. The old adage, "Only a fool has himself for a doctor," emphasizes this point.

4. It is unhealthy to make the "practice of medicine" the only interest in a physician's life.

Dedication of one's life to solving the health care needs of others is admirable. But when that becomes the only purpose, it crosses the threshold of normalcy. Distractions allow for a redress of judgment and objectivity. In the 1950s, it was reported that the average lifespan for rural general practitioners was fifty-five years because medicine *was* their life. The recent attention to limitation of "resident" work hours addresses this same concern.

5. When the workday is completed, physicians must remember that, if they are fortunate, they have loved ones waiting for them at home!

Conclusion

All axioms listed in this book are subject to interpretation. However, there are consistencies that run through all of them. First is that being a physician is not just making the correct diagnosis and prescribing the right therapy. It is about connecting with patients. Second, physicians must always be their patients' advocates. And finally, individual physicians cannot totally divorce themselves from the rest of their community.

Bibliography

1. Percival, Thomas. *Medical Ethics, A Code of Institutes and Precepts, Adapted to the Professional Conduct of Physicians and Surgeons.* S. Russell, Strand London, 1803.
2. *Code of Medical Ethics. Current Opinions and Annotations, 2012–2013 ed.* American Medical Association, Council on Ethical and Judicial Affairs, Chicago, Illinois.
3. Feldman L. S., Block 1., 'Common Courtesy' Lacking Among Doctors-in-Training, *Johns Hopkins Medicine*, 10/23/13.
4. Kohn, Linda T., Corrigan, Janet M., and Donaldson, Molla S. *To Err Is Human: Building a Safer Health Care System.* Washington, DC: Institute of Medicine, National Academy Press, 1999.
5. Lazare, Aaron. *On Apology.* Oxford University Press, 2004.
6. Meldrum, Helen. *Characteristics of Compassion: Portraits of Exemplary Physicians.* Jones and Bartlett Publishers, 2010.
7. Tenery, R. *In Search of Medicine's Moral Compass.* Brown Books Publishing, Dallas, Texas, 2011.
8. Osler, William. *Aequanimitas: With Other Addresses to Medical Students, Nurses and Practitioners of Medicine*, 3rd ed. P. Blakeston's Son & Co., Philadelphia, Pennsylvania, 1932. N.B. A gift to all medical school graduates from Eli Lilly and Company in 1935.

www.ingramcontent.com/pod-product-compliance
Lightning Source LLC
Chambersburg PA
CBHW021415170526
45164CB00002B/660